TABLE OF CONTENTS

I0412440

INTRODUCTION

Many people struggle with losing weight. They spend a lot of time, effort and money getting down to their desired goal only to regain every pound they lost. A while later, they try again. What happened? How can you lose weight and keep it off? The answer lies in how you view weight loss. Think of weight loss as a steady stream of easy lifestyle changes you make. Each change brings you one step closer to your desired goal. Because you adjust your lifestyle habits, this weight loss will last forever. You will never have to repeat this work again.

When you are ready to begin your final weight loss journey, pick up this book and start your success story. The book is loaded with no nonsense, practical tips that are proven to help you shred pounds. This is the same advice I have given nearly 3,000 families in over 25 years of running a weight control program. Data collected from the program suggests that when these tips are followed, you can lose weight. I have simplified these tips because I know that you lead busy, stressful lives. You just want to know what to do to lose weight and you want real, honest information that works. Start with the first chapter, incorporate the change into your life, and when you feel ready move on to the next tip. There is no particular time frame for implementing these changes because everyone's weight loss journey is different. The important thing is to master each tip as you make your way through the book. After a while, these changes will become automatic habits and just a normal part of your everyday life. Pretty soon you will look back and realize you are not the same person you were when you began this journey. You know too much now to ever go back to your old ways. As you take care of the changes you are making, the weight loss will follow. Enjoy the ride.

Carmen Mikhail, PhD

1. REASONS FOR LOSING WEIGHT

Brainstorm all the reasons you have for losing weight. Start a journal that you will keep in a safe place and write down these reasons on the first page of the journal. Perhaps you want to be healthier. Maybe you want to control your high cholesterol, high blood pressure, diabetes, or low back pain. Possibly you want to have more energy to run around with your children or participate in sports. You may wish to look better or fit into a favorite outfit or bathing suit. Weight loss may also help you feel better about yourself and be more positive about your life. Perhaps you want to fit into an airplane seat, movie theater seat, or stadium seat at the game. You might also feel that weight loss will improve your intimacy with a loved one. The more you have an idea of what weight loss will contribute to your life the more you will be able to stay on track. Read through your list of reasons for weight loss often to help yourself stay on track with your program.

2. ARE YOU READY?

Take time to evaluate whether you are ready, willing and able to lose weight at this time in your life. Make sure your reasons for losing weight are compelling enough and outweigh any potential barriers you may have to staying on track. What is your current level of motivation for sticking to a lifestyle change even when things get tough? Do you have some things in your life that you need to take care of before embarking on this program? For example, are your relationships and financial situation relatively stable? Although there will never be a perfect time to start a weight control program it would help if you picked a time when life was not so complicated. Do you have any addictions such as smoking or alcohol abuse you need to take care of before losing weight? Is there any particular reason you want to lose weight at this time in your life? If you can see yourself making some new changes for the next several weeks no matter how hard life gets you are most likely ready to start a weight control program.

3. SET A WEIGHT GOAL

Set a realistic weight goal. You don't need a weight table for
this, just a few minutes to sit down and be honest with yourself.
Think about a weight that you were comfortable at in the past 10
years or so. Then write this down as a 5-pound weight range
rather than as one single weight. There is evidence that losing
even 10% of your body weight can result in improvement to your
health. Keep in mind that taking weight off slowly gives you the
best chance to maintain your weight loss. Aim for a weight loss
of 1 to 2 pounds per week. To do this you'll need to burn 500 to
1,000 calories more than what you consume each day. If you
want to lose a lot of weight, say more than 20 pounds, pick
several smaller weight goals to avoid feeling overwhelmed. Now
that you've selected your weight goal set your daily focus more
on your behavior changes rather than on the weight. The final
weight is the destination but what's much more important is the
journey, all the changes that you will make every day to stay on
track. If you focus on these changes the weight loss will follow.

4. TAKE A PICTURE OF YOURSELF/ START WEIGHT CHART

Ask a friend or family member to take a "before" picture of you. Try to take it facing the camera from head to toe. It also may be a good idea to take a picture facing sideways. Be brave since this may be hard to do. Tape these photos in your journal. Leave room for at least a few "after" pictures that you can proudly display in the future. Whenever you need encouragement you can refer to these pictures and compare them to what you now look like in the mirror. Start a chart in which you will record your weight. Don't forget to write down your starting weight. After that it is necessary to weigh yourself only once per week. You can use a graph to show your progress or simply list your weekly weights. Try to weigh yourself at the same time and day each week, perhaps first thing on a Monday morning to keep you on track all weekend. If you like you can also record your weekly chest/bust, waist and hip measurements to give yourself an extra pat on the back for your progress as you go along.

5. START A FOOD AND ACTIVITY RECORD

One of the best ways to change your behavior is to start recording the actions that you want to change. Start keeping a record of all that you eat. Write down the amount and kind of food you eat, making sure to include everything that goes into your mouth. Don't forget to write down everything you drink as well. It's also very helpful to record the time you ate, who was there, what you were doing and how you were feeling during eating. When you look back at your food records you may notice some situations or feelings that cause you to overeat. You also will want to keep track of your physical activity. Record exercise as well as anything you do to move, such as walking up stairs or walking at the mall. Records can be kept in a notebook, calendar or anywhere that works for you. Try to record your food intake and physical activity right after eating and doing an activity.

6. INCREASE YOUR PHYSICAL ACTIVITY

Start increasing your physical activity. Think of all the benefits to exercise such as losing fat and gaining muscle, keeping your heart healthy, reducing stress, sleeping better, staying mentally alert, increasing your energy level, having a more mobile and flexible body, and living longer. The easiest way to start right now is to walk more often. Buy an activity tracker which measures your steps or use an app on your smartphone, and record the daily steps in your journal or calendar. Make sure you have a comfortable pair of walking shoes and socks. If you're not sure where to start, take your average daily step count for seven days and aim to increase it by no more than 10% each week. So, if you walked 15 minutes per day last week you can walk 16 ½ minutes per day this week (adding 10% or 1 ½ minutes) and so on. Do some easy stretches before you start. You can walk anywhere at all: a nearby park or field, a shopping mall, a trail, up and down hallways at home or work, or in your neighborhood. It might be helpful to find some exercise buddies who will walk with you in order to stay motivated. Make sure to get medical clearance from your doctor before starting a walking program.

7. UNDERSTAND WEIGHT GAIN

People with weight issues are really not eating much more than those who are normal weight. It's just that even the tiniest extra amount that you eat each day adds up over weeks, months, and years to create excess weight. A pound of excess weight comes from eating roughly 3,500 extra calories. Say you eat an extra 100 calories per day. This translates into gaining approximately an extra pound every month, or an extra 12 pounds per year. Now, it doesn't take much to consume an extra 100 calories per day. One slice of cheese, a spoon of mayonnaise, or a small glass of juice or low fat milk each contains about 100 calories. So just by adding one of these to your daily diet you will gain 12 pounds a year. It really makes you think twice about the little things that you consume on a daily basis and whether it is worth it to you to keep these in your diet. The good news is that by eliminating a few of these small food items you are well on your way to successful weight loss.

8. REARRANGE FRIDGE AND PANTRY

Go through your fridge and pantry and make sure that tempting food is out of sight. Get rid of foods that are high in calories and fat, especially those with a lot of sugar, white flour, and salt. Instead, place healthy food at the front and center of your cupboards and fridge so this will be what you reach for when hungry. A plate of fresh cut vegetables with a light dip can be placed in the center of your fridge. Replace sugary drinks with water, sparkling water or drinks that contain less than 10 calories per eight ounce serving. Substitute a bowl of fresh fruit for candy and sweets. If you want to have a small treat every now and then, it is better to have these treats outside the home than bringing them into the house where you are more tempted to eat them often. Otherwise, keep a few lower calorie treats at home if you need a little something special. Ask other family members to help you by refraining from bringing junk food home.

9. EAT AT ONLY ONE PLACE

Start eating all your meals and snacks at only one place in your home, seated at the dining or kitchen table. Eliminate eating at other places at home, for example in the living room or bedroom in front of the TV or while on a tablet, or while driving. The more that you eat in several places the more those places become associated with eating. You need to wipe out any association with eating other than at a dining or kitchen table. This also makes you more aware of what you are eating because it eliminates eating while distracted. Have your family eat dinner together nearly every day since family dinners are often associated with making healthier choices. When you come to eat, serve yourself at the stovetop and then take only your plate to the table. Leave all the remaining food in the kitchen area so it is not visible when you are eating at the table. This may help you rethink whether you really wanted that second helping or if you were reaching for more food simply because it was conveniently placed right in front of you at the table.

10. NOTICE EATING PATTERNS

Look back at your food records and notice if there are certain situations or times when you are more likely to eat. Perhaps you eat more when you are bored, upset, hurt, or angry. You may eat more late at night, when alone, or when you are with certain people. You also may be more likely to eat when you simply smell or see food. Becoming aware of these patterns will help you to start thinking of solutions for situations where you may eat more even though you are not really physically hungry. Write down situations that make you eat more and for each circumstance write down some other things that you can do instead. For example, if you eat in response to boredom write down a list of alternative activities such as walking at a mall, going to the park, listening to music, or calling a friend on the phone. If you eat more when you see food, try to keep all food away from sight, stored either in the fridge or pantry. Pretty soon you will be eating only when you are truly physically hungry and not in response to a lot of other situations that trigger eating.

11. A SIMPLE WAY TO FILL YOUR PLATE

When serving your plate of food a quick rule of thumb is to visualize how much space each food should occupy. Fill ½ of the plate with nonstarchy vegetables, ¼ of the plate with starches, whole grains or bread and ¼ with lean meat, poultry, fish or seafood. You may also add a cup of fat-free milk and a small piece or serving of fresh fruit to this meal. The vegetables could be cooked vegetables, salad, or any combination of vegetables you like. This method is easy to follow whether you are eating at home or eating out and does not involve elaborate calculations. Everyone in the family can grasp this concept and apply it, even children. The more you follow this way of filling your plate the more you will become accustomed to it. It will be easier to get your minimum daily intake of vegetables and fruit as well. Don't be afraid to ask for substitutions when eating out so you can stick to this method of filling your plate.

12. PLAN AHEAD FOR SPECIAL OCCASIONS

Whenever you have a social occasion coming up it will most likely involve food. Whether it is a party, dinner, church function, club meeting, shower, wedding, family reunion or other event, you need to be prepared with a game plan. Try to find out in advance what foods will be served or available and decide what you can eat that will allow you to stay on target with your plan of healthy eating. Write down in advance what you will eat and take the list with you. Arrive at the event having eaten a small snack so you are not overly hungry and tempted to break your action plan. Another strategy is to arrive after everyone has eaten. When at the event, try to focus on the social interaction and on anything else that is going on around you and stay away from the area where the food is visible. You may find that by focusing on everything other than the food your experience of the event will be much more rewarding and enriching.

13. SLOW DOWN YOUR EATING

Eat slowly and chew your food properly. Why should you do this? It takes about 20 minutes from the time you start eating for your stomach to signal to your brain that you are full. If you eat rapidly you may not realize that you've eaten enough until you have overeaten. You can do a lot of caloric damage in 20 minutes. How do you slow down your eating? Put down your fork and knife, or sandwich, between every bite. Take smaller bites of food. Eat with chopsticks. Give yourself a 2-minute break in the middle of your meal. Savor your food and really enjoy its taste and smell. Drink small sips of water between bites. You can also put on some soft music and light a few candles to create a peaceful ambience at dinnertime. Get good conversations going so that everyone around the table also slows down their eating. That way you will not feel so rushed. As an incentive to keep eating slowly remind yourself that the slowest eater at the table is often the slimmest person.

14. SET WEEKLY GOALS

Set weekly goals for changing your behavior. You could set a goal to change some aspect of your eating. Examples are slowing down your eating, eating only at the table, turning off TV during mealtimes, or keeping a food record. Alternately, you could set a goal involving physical activity, such as walking a certain amount of time 5 times per week, or trying a new activity in the next week. It is better to target your behavior than weight change when setting goals since your weight may fluctuate due to many factors whereas you are always in control of your behavior. Make sure that you also set a reward for reaching your behavior goal. You can put together a contract for yourself where you write down your goal and reward, possibly posting this on your fridge. When aiming for weight loss it helps to break everything down into smaller, more manageable behavioral steps and reward yourself every step of the way.

15. ASK FOR HELP

Enlist the help of others in your quest for a healthier lifestyle. Don't be afraid to ask for assistance instead of always being the one looking after everyone else's needs. You may need loved ones to help you by keeping your home free of unhealthy foods, joining you in exercising, supporting and encouraging your efforts, or doing anything else that you feel would be useful. Ask friends and family members to show love for you with rewards other than food. Remember to say no to food pushers or those who sabotage your diet. Try to interact more with those around you who choose to live healthier lifestyles since this may inspire you and keep you on track. Being assertive – asking for what you need and want – will send out a signal to others and reaffirm to yourself how important you are as a person and how much you deserve to look after yourself.

16. AVOID FAD DIETS

Fad diets get you started on a vicious cycle of losing and gaining weight that can be unmotivating, unhealthy and even dangerous. They usually focus on a combination of foods or ask you to eliminate food groups altogether. People who make unrealistic claims and dramatic statements about expected results often back these diets. They often sell pills, products, or seminars as part of their program. Fad diets offer only temporary solutions and do not help you with long-term weight control. Once stopped, you will usually regain the weight quickly. The best program is one that focuses on weight loss of no more than two pounds per week, and includes a varied diet with moderate portions of healthy food and increased physical activity. Even though you are desperate to lose weight don't be tempted to do something that doesn't feel right. If it sounds too good to be true it probably is.

17. LISTEN TO YOUR BODY

Learn to really listen to how your body is feeling to determine whether you are truly physically hungry. If you are hungry your stomach may growl or feel empty, you might feel weak, light-headed, faint, or tired, or you may get a headache. Become familiar with your own body cues that signal physical hunger, and write these down or at least make a mental note of them. Now distinguish these from cues that signal you to eat when you are "emotionally" hungry, such as boredom, depression, anger, stress, anxiety, or the sight and smell of food. In order to stay on track with weight loss you need to eat only when physically hungry. If you're not sure if you're really hungry, set a kitchen timer to go off in 20 minutes and if at that time you're still hungry go ahead and eat.

18. STOP EATING WHEN FULL

This is simple advice yet sometimes challenging to follow. The minute you feel satisfied stop eating, put your fork and knife down, and leave the table. If you are concerned about not wasting food pack the rest in a container or if you are eating out ask for a to-go box. Don't worry about the fact that millions of people all over the world are going hungry. If you clean your plate you are not helping them one bit. Try to ignore conditioning you may have received as a child that you must finish everything on your plate. If you consistently eat to the point of feeling uncomfortably full you, address issues that are causing you to stuff your feelings inside with food. Go over food records and your journal to understand what emotions trigger you to overeat in this manner.

19. PAY ATTENTION TO SELF TALK

Become aware of the thoughts about weight loss that you often have. Some of these may be negative and very discouraging such as believing that you won't be able to stay on track with your eating and exercise plan or being hard on yourself if you slip. Replace these with more positive statements that emphasize your ability to stay on track and work hard to change your lifestyle. Remember that the thoughts you have are powerful determinants of what eventually happens to you. If you see yourself going down a successful path then most likely you will succeed. That is why it is so important to always keep positive thoughts and expectations in your head and throw out the negative thoughts into an imaginary trashcan in your mind. If you learn to change your thinking and be supportive of yourself then your behavior will follow.

20. EAT MORE UNPROCESSED FOOD

Eat a large proportion of your food in its most natural, unrefined form possible, in other words the way it occurs in nature. Unprocessed food will fill you up but often is not as fattening as processed food. Examples of natural, unprocessed foods include fresh vegetables and fruit, whole grains, beans, lentils, and fresh fish or chicken. Most unprocessed food can be found at the outer borders of a grocery store whereas the processed food is usually found in the center of the store. You can tell a food is processed if it comes in a box, bag, can, carton, jar or bottle. Such foods often have extra ingredients such as white sugar or unhealthy fats added to enhance their flavor, increasing their caloric content. A good rule of thumb is that if the food has a food label it is most likely a processed food and you would benefit from finding a more natural, unrefined alternative.

21. WHAT ARE YOU DRINKING?

Pay attention to the caloric content of what you are drinking all day. You may be eating a relatively healthy diet but drinking a lot of sugary drinks that are contributing significantly to your daily caloric intake without realizing it. For example, orange juice, low-fat chocolate milk, vanilla soymilk, or some energy drinks are packed with more calories than regular soda yet most people think they are making a healthy choice when drinking these beverages. Try to get used to drinking water when thirsty. If you need some flavor add some fresh lemon slices or mint leaves. You also may make some black or herb tea with teabags and water, and serve over ice. If you absolutely must have a sweetener, try decreasing the amount of your sweetener by 10% each week until you can enjoy the tea without any sweetener at all. Remember to write down all your drinks in your food record so you can become more aware of just how many calories you are drinking as well as eating.

22. WHAT'S EATING YOU?

There's a popular saying that when it comes to weight control it's not what you're eating but what's eating you. Look deep down for underlying emotional feelings that may be triggering you to overeat. Take some quiet time for yourself and really think hard about this. You can talk with a trusted loved one if necessary. You could also journal about this till you get to the bottom of what's bothering you that's causing you to turn to food for what you really need. Some people use food for emotional reasons or for avoiding having to deal with painful issues. If this is you, ask yourself "If I weren't stuffing my feelings with food right now what would I be feeling?" Until you get to the root of the problem you may find yourself going around in circles, so do whatever you need to do to resolve these underlying issues and heal yourself. This could be a big step in developing a more healthy relationship with food.

23. MAKE EXERCISE EASY

Arrange everything so it is easy to exercise every day. Take out your old exercise equipment that has been sitting in the garage or attic, dust it off, and put it right in front of the TV in the living room. If you drive to work keep a gym bag in your car with everything you will need to go directly to the gym before or after work. Don't forget to pack a gadget with your favorite music to keep you going during workouts. If you plan on exercising outdoors develop a backup plan in case of bad weather. Set up regular times to work out with your exercise buddies and stick to them. Put together an agreement in which the person missing a scheduled exercise session must pay the other one a significant sum of money or do a chore for them such as washing his or her car. Turn off your smartphone so you can focus on your exercise and avoid distractions. Vary your routine and choose something you really like to do so you will be more likely to stay on track with your exercise plan.

24. DINING OUT

Order baked, grilled or steamed entrees with nutritious side dishes such as steamed vegetables. Refrain from cream sauces or dishes baked with cheese. Fish or seafood will usually be your healthiest choices, so browse this section of the menu first followed by chicken and then beef, pork or lamb. Don't be afraid to specify how you want your food prepared. Ask for sauces and dressings to be served on the side. Skip the bread basket. Instead, start your meal with a salad made with fresh, wholesome vegetables. Avoid cheese, bacon bits or croutons on the salad. Most restaurants serve large portions so split a portion or ask for a "to go" box at the beginning of the meal and place half your entrée in it before you start eating. Ask the waiter to refrain from bringing the dessert tray to your table. Remember that eating out is not an excuse to eat any differently than you would at home. What to order for dessert? Nearly every restaurant should be able to provide you with a bowl of fresh berries in season.

25. INVOLVE THE ENTIRE FAMILY

Involve your spouse and children in your weight control efforts. It is never too early to start teaching your children healthy eating habits. Contrary to popular belief your overweight children will not grow out of their condition unless you change their lifestyle. The longer your children are overweight during childhood the greater their chances of remaining overweight as adults. In fact, this generation of children is predicted not to live as long as their parents because of the problem of childhood obesity. Set some goals for the entire family such as eating meals together at the table with the TV, tablets and smartphones off, or eating fast food only once per week. Then set individual goals for each family member depending on what they need to do to get on track. Make sure to include children in all active chores such as vacuuming the house or walking the dog. The more the entire family changes its lifestyle the greater the chance of success in all members. While you're at it, modify your pet's lifestyle to be healthier so they don't miss out on the action.

26. WORK ON DEVELOPING CONFIDENCE

The more you think like a confident person the easier weight loss will be. People who are confident believe in themselves and their ability to get the job done. They also take good care of themselves because they believe they are worth it. They do not put anything in their life on hold until they reach a certain weight but realize they deserve the best that life has to offer everyday, unconditionally, regardless of their weight. That includes the outfit that you have been dying to buy or the relationship that you want to go for. How do you develop confidence? Start by acting "as if". Wake up one morning and act your entire day "as if" you had unlimited confidence. Walk in the center of the hallway, greet people by looking them in the eye, hold your head up high, stand in the center of the elevator, smile at everyone, and wear something special. How does it feel? Would you mind repeating it again day after day?

27. TRICK YOUR EYE

Serve your meals on small plates and bowls so it will appear as though your entire plate is full of food. Likewise, use smaller glasses when drinking. Check the size of your utensils and if necessary replace them with smaller forks, knives and spoons. Soon you will get used to the size of the new plates and utensils. Make sure that you always eat from a plate and not a container. If you eat from a deep container such as a to-go box, bag or ice cream tub it hides the actual amount you are eating. Decorate the food on your plate with garnishes such as a sprig of parsley or a slice of lemon. Restaurant portions are nearly always larger than necessary and served on large plates, and "super sized" portions can be large enough for two or three people. Therefore, when eating out ask for a healthy appetizer that will usually come served on a smaller plate.

28. HANDLING SLIPS

Do your best to avoid situations that get you in trouble with food. For example, avoid buffet restaurants that may encourage you to overeat once you see all the food. Keep tempting snacks out of sight at home. Better yet, don't even bring the food home. If you need a treat, just go out and eat it rather than having constant access to it. If you do slip and eat more than planned don't be too hard on yourself or engage in a lot of negative self-talk such as "Well I slipped up now, I may as well keep eating". Just treat the next minute as the start of the rest of your program and gently remind yourself that you can make better choices at the next meal. Most people take a few steps backward every now and then. It's how you choose to handle the situation that will really get you back on track. Success is never accomplished without a few setbacks along the way.

29. EAT TO LIVE

Do you eat to live or live to eat? Practice eating to live and focus on food mostly for physical nourishment. Think of food simply as fuel and replenish your body the same way you would stop for gas only when the gas tank in your car is empty. Do you ever catch yourself living to eat? For example, are you paying too much attention to food, constantly thinking about the next meal or thinking about food when you are not around it? Practice living in the moment and enjoying what is currently happening around you. Focus especially on the other small things in life that bring you joy such as meaningful relationships or activities. When you find other things in your life that give you emotional satisfaction, you won't have to use food as an outlet for your needs. If you catch yourself thinking about food ask yourself if you are truly hungry or just need an emotional boost. Then do what you need to take care of your emotional needs.

30. FOOD SHOPPING

Before going grocery shopping, prepare a list of healthy foods that you need. This will make it easier to stick to the list once you are actually in the store and are tempted by other foods. Preplan your meals so you have healthy choices for breakfast, lunch, dinner and a snack. Make sure to shop after eating since you will make better food choices when you are not hungry. Allow yourself enough time to read food labels or consider healthier alternatives before putting food items in your cart. Consider leaving your children at home so they won't ask for unhealthy foods such as sugary cereals that are often placed at a child's eye level on the shelves. Buy most of your food from the produce, dairy, fish and poultry sections of the store. Plan on eating at least 5 to 7 servings of vegetables or fruit daily and buy accordingly. Make sure to stock up on water and avoid sugary drinks and juice. A good start to making wise choices is keeping the right kinds of food around in the first place.

31. STAY ON TRACK

Post a picture of yourself at a desirable weight at eye level on your fridge. Imagine yourself already at that weight and think of that image on a daily basis. What are you doing? How are you feeling? Journaling may help you answer these questions. Imagine the lifestyle you are following in order to stay at that desirable weight. Put together a list of specific things you are doing with your behavior, diet and exercise. Now write down some of these on post-it notes and place them around your picture on the fridge. The notes could provide you with tips that are important for you. For example, "get up during commercial break", "avoid eating after dinner", "take Lucky for a walk". You can also add some stop signs alongside statements such as "Do I really need this?" "Nothing tastes as good as being skinny feels" or "A moment on the lips, a lifetime on the hips".

32. MAKE HEALTHY FOODS MORE APPETIZING

Try out new recipes and experiment with new ways of putting healthy meal ingredients together. Instead of buying the same fruit and vegetables add some exotic varieties such as papayas or fresh fennel. Add some fresh herbs such as dill to salmon or basil to salad. Better yet, grow your own herbs in your garden or flowerpot so they are available whenever you need to enhance the flavor of your food. Learn to use spices, herbs, garlic, onions, ground pepper, mustard, or capers for a virtually calorie free way of making food delicious. Adding fresh lemon or lime to foods such as fish, chicken or vegetables is another great way to add zest. Make a low-calorie vegetable dip by adding some dry onion soup mix to low-fat plain yogurt. Still not sure how to put healthy food together? Why not purchase a healthy cookbook or sign up for healthy cooking classes?

33. SAVE TIME IN PREPARING HEALTHY MEALS

Are you feeling that there's not enough time to shop or cook healthy meals? Consider having your groceries delivered or purchasing your food through an Internet grocery shopping service, if available in your area. You'll still come out ahead financially than if you ate out. Another alternative is to keep some healthy frozen dinners available to use when necessary. While heating them up you can prepare a simple green salad as your side dish. You can also fix some meals on weekends and simply heat them up during the week. You might even cook extra so the food lasts over several mealtimes. Most grocery stores have a whole rotisserie chicken available for pickup in the prepared foods section that could be paired with a bag of salad greens and whole grain buns for an easy meal. For a quick fix, have a pizza prepared with fresh vegetables delivered to your home. Make sure to skip the extra cheese.

34. EAT WHAT YOU WANT

It seems counterintuitive to eat what you really want but in the end this may give you more psychological satisfaction. Say you want ice cream. You won't allow yourself any and so you get frozen yogurt instead. You get a large serving and add a topping so you won't feel that deprived. By the time you add up all the calories consumed, you may as well have had what you really wanted in the first place, a serving of ice cream. It would have prevented you from going around in circles trying to fill in the gap with something else that wasn't that satisfying and most probably ended up having nearly as many calories. By eating moderate portions of what you really want you may be able to stop when you are full because in your mind you know you can have that food whenever you want. It is always our nature to want what we cannot have so we must trick ourselves into thinking that we can have whatever we want whenever we want it. That way we won't really want it very often.

35. LIMITED FOOD BUDGET

Use beans and lentils instead of meat for protein. Otherwise, a whole chicken is often a good buy. You could roast it one day and use leftovers for sandwiches and salads the next. Check to see which foods are on sale before going through the grocery store. You could buy some foods in bulk, as long as it will not cause you to overeat. Purchase foods in co-ops or at the farmer's market. Most ethnic food stores have good deals, such as corn tortillas at the local Mexican market. Replace expensive salad dressings with a little olive oil and vinegar. Buy vegetables and fruits in season to save money. Some frozen fruit is cheaper than fresh fruit and does not go bad, so there is no waste. Replace costly soda with water. Low-cost meals include whole-wheat pasta with vegetables, beans and rice with salad, or a rice and vegetable stir-fry. Try bulk oatmeal for breakfast. Of course, eating less also saves you money.

36. WEIGHT GAIN

Sit down with a pen and paper and write down times in your life that were associated with weight gain. It could be the start of school or a job, time after loss of a loved one, divorce, job stress, or family problems. Reflect and journal about how you were really feeling during those events. What were you hoping food would do for you at those times? Now write about how you can take care of yourself emotionally in the future if times get tough. Who can you lean on for support? How can you soothe yourself in ways that don't involve food? You can call close friends or family members, or reach out to members of your church. Soothe yourself by getting a massage or manicure, playing a round of golf, watching a great movie, buying yourself some fresh flowers, playing with your pet, listening to great music, meditating, having a long candle-lit bubble bath, going to your favorite escape for the weekend, going for a long walk, dancing to great music, or anything else that makes you feel happy.

37. BENEFITS OF BEING HEAVY

It seems counterproductive but sometimes people hold on to the benefits of being heavy. For example, being large can be used as an excuse for not moving on with your life, goals, or relationships. You can put things on hold, assuring yourself that you will get to them once you have lost weight. If you have issues surrounding physical intimacy being heavy can protect you from being in a situation where you have to deal with them. Are you punishing yourself for something that happened a long time ago that you should forgive yourself for? You may be hiding underneath what you perceive to be the protective layers of being overweight. Ask yourself what your life would be like if you lost the weight. Is there anything you would have to face that you currently fear? The more you deal with these things the more that you can finally make peace with your body once and for all and move on to the healthy lifestyle you deserve.

38. MAKE FRIENDS WITH YOUR BODY

Learn to love the body you have. Accept the fact that there is no such thing as a perfect body, even at the right weight. When pictures are taken of models, several hundred shots are taken in order to come up with the one shot that makes the model look near perfect. Even then his or her body is often air brushed and other alterations are made. Don't buy into the illusion that you have to look the way people in a magazine look. If you met them on the street they wouldn't even look perfect. So you're putting pressure on yourself to look a certain way that realistically doesn't even exist. Just focus on getting to a healthy weight for yourself and accept your body shape. Learn to look in a mirror and focus on what you really like about your looks rather than on what is wrong with your body. Surprisingly, you'll soon see a nice looking person in the mirror in front of you.

39. YOU CONTROL YOUR WEIGHT

Recognize that the ability to control your weight resides within you and nowhere else. Slight modifications in your metabolic rate or genetic makeup, or side effects of medication do not dictate your ultimate weight. Your doctor may be able to provide advice but he or she does not control your weight. Fast food outlets may be everywhere and TV commercials promoting junk food are abundant, yet they do not have power over your weight. The government may be trying to educate the public about the perils of obesity but it is not in charge of your personal weight. Life circumstances may be difficult and extremely trying at times, but you have a choice about how ultimately they affect your weight. In the end you are the one who owns your body and takes care of it. You have complete freedom and also responsibility for looking after this most precious gift.

40. EVALUATE PAST SUCCESSES

Think about past times you have worked on losing weight. What do you remember as being the most effective components of your program? Everyone is different and sometimes things that worked for others may not necessarily work for you. If you can make a list of things that worked for you in the past you can use this as a guide for what methods to keep using. Likewise, if you know certain methods have not worked for you in the past, stay away from these. Some people do well working on their own while others need the support of a group or an exercise buddy. Some prefer pre-packaged meals whereas others want to cook for themselves. Some people want to focus mostly on increasing exercise. Evaluate your preferences and lifestyle and tailor your plan to fit these. There is no right or wrong way to lose weight. The important thing is that it works for you.

41. MAKE A LONG-TERM COMMITMENT

Look at your weight control program as a permanent lifestyle change rather than as a diet. If you believe you are on a "diet" you may start to feel deprived and that feeling of deprivation often leads to bingeing and sneaking food. However, if you aim for slow, steady changes for the rest of your life you will stay on track. Before you know it you will have followed new ways of eating and exercising and you will start to see improvements in how you look and feel. Recognize that there will never be a food you need to eliminate from your diet completely. For example, if you absolutely love chocolate you can still have it occasionally in moderate amounts. Actually, it's important for you to schedule an occasional treat so you don't end up feeling too deprived. Making a commitment to slow, steady behavior changes will get you further in terms of weight control than making extreme changes for only a short time.

42. EMOTIONAL HUNGER

We often eat when we feel emotional hunger. We may crave certain comfort foods, often sweet and rich, that we used to placate feelings in the past. Some of these behaviors and patterns may have been shaped in childhood when parents or caretakers gave you food to soothe you. It is time to recognize that food will never be an effective solution for negative feelings. We can eat all we want but in the end the feelings that triggered the eating will still be there, waiting to be resolved. The only way to deal with negative feelings is to acknowledge them for what they are, journal about them, or talk to a good friend or family member about your struggles. Even a good cry will often do the job. Think of times in the past when you ate in response to emotional hunger. Now go back and write down some alternative ways that you could deal with these feelings in the future. It is possible to rewire our brains so we select better ways of dealing with emotions from now on.

43. MORE STRATEGIES FOR FOOD SHOPPING

Purchase a wide variety of healthy foods. Keep trying new items that you can incorporate into your diet. Give the regular items you always purchase a break for a week. Buy small servings of food and small pieces of fresh fruit. Large food quantities invite overeating. You are more likely to serve yourself a hefty portion of low-fat ice cream if you dip into a huge container rather than a small one. Keep away from parts of the store that tempt you, for example, the bakery. Buy foods that are not already prepared. If you have a lot of ready to eat food at home you may be more tempted to take it out and eat it for a snack. Purchase foods that take a long time to eat, for example, boiled shrimp with the shells on. Buy foods in controlled portions so you cannot have second helpings. For example, purchase only one piece of chicken and one potato for each member of the family. Reward yourself for making healthy choices at the grocery store with a bouquet of flowers.

44. PAY ATTENTION TO FOOD PORTIONS

If we don't write down our food portions in a food record we have a tendency to underestimate how much we have eaten. Therefore, it is important to continue to write down how much you have eaten every day. Become familiar with standard serving sizes and how many "servings per container" there are for most foods. For example, food labels list a half-cup of rice or pasta as one serving. You may need to measure some foods at first until you can estimate sizes. A meat serving should be no larger than the size of the palm of your hand. Unfortunately, food portions have gotten much larger in the past few years so we cannot rely on the restaurant industry to dictate normal serving sizes for us. Remember if you are super sizing your meal you are also super sizing your waistline. If you are served a larger food portion you will tend to eat it so be mindful of what constitutes a normal serving and start with only this amount.

45. HIDDEN CALORIES IN A MENU

When selecting food from a restaurant menu the terms can be confusing. Here is a list of foods to avoid ordering: Foods with 'Alfredo', 'béarnaise', 'hollandaise', or 'carbonara' sauces are high in fat. Instead, order a tomato sauce. If a food is 'creamed', 'scalloped' or served 'au gratin' or 'parmesan' it is also loaded with fats. Foods that are 'stuffed' are often stuffed with high calorie items. Avoid foods that are described with terms such as 'nuggets', 'tenders', 'popcorn', 'tempura', 'fingers', 'battered', 'breaded', 'hush puppies', or 'wonton' since these are usually deep-fried. Stay away from foods that are 'glazed', 'bacon-wrapped' or served with a 'Ranch' dressing. A quiche may seem like a good choice but the pastry is high in fat. High fat means high calories. Instead, order foods that are steamed, baked, broiled, poached or roasted. Write out the terms on this page and take them with you the next time you eat out. Congratulations, you just saved yourself loads of calories!

46. SOCIAL SUPPORT

Evaluate your relationships to make sure you get support for your healthy lifestyle. Do you have people around you who motivate you to stay on track? If not, consider starting a support group with others who want to lose weight. Telling someone else about your goals to lose weight makes you more accountable for your behavior and therefore helps you stay on track. You can call or e-mail a weight loss buddy once a week to report how you're doing. If you exercise with a partner there's a sense of responsibility to show up whenever and wherever you decided to exercise. Studies have shown that the more social support a person receives the more weight they lose in a program. They are also more successful at keeping the weight off. Therefore, recruit friends, family members, neighbors or colleagues to join you. Form a group name, get group t-shirts and set a group goal for weight loss. You'll end up having much more fun along the way.

47. MODERATION, MODERATION, MODERATION

When you decide to lose weight you can jump in too intensely and go overboard at times. However, if you cut back too much on your food intake you will end up lowering your metabolism as your body tries to adjust to its starvation mode. Slowly and steadily wins the race. Continue to aim for no more than a one or two pound weight loss per week. Think of your program as a lifestyle change rather than a diet. Don't be tempted to skip meals as a method of weight control. It only backfires, leaving you starving and setting you up for a binge later in the day. Exercise moderately and keep it varied so you don't get to a point where you are sick and tired of physical activity and want to quit. Remember, most humans cannot keep up an extreme level of intensity for a long time. It is much easier to make a commitment to moderate, reasonable lifestyle changes and goals that are achievable. Remember the fable of the tortoise and the hare? Be the tortoise.

48. USE THE INTERNET

The internet can provide you with resources for healthy eating and exercise. Join a chat group to compare weight control strategies and share success stories. Social media can be a good source of support late at night when you feel like snacking and it's too late to contact family and friends. Start a blog to post information about your own progress and how you achieved it. Make use of an online calorie counter to educate yourself about the caloric costs of eating certain foods. Some online diet programs allow you to enter your daily food intake and then calculate your calorie, fat, carbohydrate, vitamin and mineral levels. Some programs even come with a version for your smartphone. Use reliable fitness web sites for fitness information and advice. Using the internet provides you with a more flexible schedule since it is basically available 24 hours per day. Now you have no excuse not to stay on track.

49. MINIMIZE YOUR REFINED SUGAR INTAKE

Think of foods and drinks you consume regularly that contain sugar. Start with beverages such as soda, sweetened tea, fruit drinks, juice, coffee drinks, or alcoholic beverages. You'd be amazed at how many processed foods also contain sugar. Check the labels of ketchup, salad dressing, sauce, pickles, peanut butter, flavored soymilk or almond milk, and canned savory items such as spaghetti, baked beans, vegetables, and soup. The sugar may be disguised as fructose, corn syrup, sucrose, glucose, dextrose, maltose, maltodextrin, or cane juice. Sometimes if an item is fat-free it contains even more sweeteners for flavor. Foods and beverages that contain sugar are often high in calories. Furthermore, sugar is a very addictive substance. Eating sugar eventually lowers your blood sugar level, which makes you want to eat more. White starches that turn to sugar quickly in the body, such as white bread or pasta, also have the same effect. Gradually minimize your intake of these foods and you're one step closer to controlling your weight.

50. LISTEN TO MIND TALK

Tell yourself you won't be able to do something and you won't. It's called a 'self-fulfilling prophecy'. You will do whatever your thoughts are expecting you to do. If you expect to fail then you will. If you expect to succeed then you will. Therefore, expect you will be able to stay on track with your program. Look at how far you have already come and all the lifestyle changes you have made. Write them down on a piece of paper and give yourself credit for every single one. Look at the results in terms of weight change, the way clothing now fits you, your increased energy level, how much better you feel about yourself, health improvements, or any other results you have noticed. Expect that you will continue to make improvements to your diet and exercise habits and that it will get easier over time. Share this expectation with your closest friends and family members who you know will support you and believe in you. Congratulations on your continued success.

51. GET ENOUGH SLEEP

Studies have shown that people who get enough sleep weigh less than those who don't. Sleep deprivation causes hormone changes that increase hunger and decrease your body's ability to feel satisfied after eating. Additionally, if you have a good night's sleep you will feel more like exercising than if you are chronically tired. You also may rely less on sweet or starchy foods to stay awake. The more rested you feel the better you can manage stress so you won't turn to food for comfort. What can you do to sleep better? Exercise regularly but not too close to bedtime, skip sugary foods, wake up at the same time each day, and take a warm bath or practice a relaxing routine at bedtime. Some overweight individuals suffer from sleep apnea, a condition where you stop breathing for very short periods during sleep, possibly resulting in sleep deprivation. The good news is that sleep apnea improves with even modest weight loss, yet one more reason to stay on track with your healthy lifestyle.

52. TAKE CONTROL OF YOUR EATING

Eat food only when you can sit and enjoy it slowly. Avoid eating in a hurry. Identify high-risk places such as bakeries or candy stores and detour around them. When you eat, leave some food on your plate so you get into the habit of not always cleaning your plate. Take a healthy lunch to work so you are not tempted to eat out. Pack school lunches and healthy snacks for your children so they do not eat the foods offered at school which usually are high in calories and low in nutrition. Put leftovers into separate portion sized containers so you have the correct amount of food when you reach for leftovers. When eating out don't be afraid or embarrassed to ask for a kid's sized meal. You can even get it to go. Remember to not bring fattening food into the house. The more you see it the more likely you are to eat it. One last way to control your eating is to drink a full glass of water before your meal. Otherwise, take sips of water between bites. Keep practicing these behaviors and soon they will solidify into habits.

53. MAKE FRIENDS WITH YOUR SCALE

Get on a weigh scale only once per week rather than daily. If you find that you are weighing yourself more often than this put your scale in a less visible place. You can measure your progress by the fit of your clothing rather than getting into a power struggle with your weigh scale. As you exercise and get fit you develop muscle, which weighs more than fat. Therefore, the pounds may not come off a rapidly as you want but you are still losing inches. If after weighing or taking your measurements once per week you find that you are getting off track, develop a realistic plan for the next week to continue with your progress. Add some fun physical activity to your routine. Go out dancing or talk a walk in a beautiful place. Remember, the scale is there to give you helpful feedback. It is for you, not against you. If you stay on track with your program, eventually your scale will reward you with a number that suggests you are moving in the right direction.

54. RESTRUCTURE YOUR COMMUNITY

Ask for healthier foods to be served at your work cafeteria and your children's schools. Request shower facilities in your place of employment so you can walk or bike to work. Attend the wellness programs offered at work. Lobby for more bike paths and fitness centers in your community. Set up a group to walk or bike to work together. Set up another one to walk or bike kids to school together. Ask your children's school to provide daily physical education, recess, and physical activity programs after school. Ask fast food chains and restaurants to develop healthier menu choices. When they do, purchase these items so their introduction will be financially feasible. Eat at restaurants designed to serve healthier foods so they will stay in business. If more community members demand facilities to help them maintain a healthier lifestyle the community will respond accordingly.

55. BEWARE OF "HEALTHY" FOODS

Food manufacturers are clever at giving us what we want. If we want to have our cake and eat it too they create "healthy" versions of the foods we crave, telling us it is fine to eat these foods since they are fat-free or low fat. However, a lot of fat-free or low fat foods are high in sugar to compensate taste-wise for the fact that they have less fat. Additionally, these foods often contain nearly as many calories as their regular fat counterparts. Often people eat more fat-free or low fat foods since they view them as being healthier, guilt-free versions of regular foods. Since these foods may not taste as good as the regular offerings we may eat more of them just to obtain the same psychological satisfaction that comes from eating regular foods. Check the labels for calories in foods such as reduced fat cookies, energy bars, desserts, smoothies, and flavored yogurt and you may be surprised at just how fattening they are.

56. LEARN TO CONTROL STRESS

Chronic stress releases hormones such as cortisol that can increase your appetite and eventually cause you to eat more. We sometimes cope with stress by snacking and the longer we do this the more that overeating becomes paired with stress. What are some healthier ways of dealing with stress? Alcohol does not help in the long run since it adds a lot of calories and impulse eating, and drinking in response to stress is another unhealthy patterned behavior. You may also want to avoid caffeine since it often contributes to that jittery feeling. You can learn some breathing and relaxation exercises and participate in calming activities. Go for a walk, get a massage, write in your journal, talk to a trusted friend, join a support group, do some yoga, listen to your favorite music, and spend time with relaxing people.

57. FOOD TRIGGERS

Go through your food records and identify patterns in your day that cause you to overeat when you're not hungry. Perhaps you're emotionally upset, bored, or feeling tired. You may also respond to the sight and smell of food, wanting to eat when you see food or see others eating it. Practice ways of resolving distress other than by turning to food. Also carry out some strategies to steer clear of food when it is visible or when others are eating. Continue to journal rather than stuffing your feelings inside. In your journal keep track of your accomplishments in choosing your new lifestyle. List down all your new behavior patterns and reflect on how far you've come. You can also write down any special statements or comments that motivate you to stay on track. Constantly encouraging yourself in this way will help you resist any food triggers that you encounter along the way.

58. HELP YOUR CHILDREN

Model a healthy lifestyle for your children so they develop good habits at an early age. The longer they remain overweight as children the greater their chances of being overweight adults. It is therefore never too early to start weight management with children. Contrary to popular belief, they will not simply grow out of it. The longer you wait the more their habits are becoming fixed. Encourage all your children to adopt a healthy lifestyle rather than singling out only those with a weight problem. Introduce them slowly to healthy foods and reward them for trying. Be positive about making good choices so they can adopt this attitude. Involve children in meal planning, and in shopping for and preparing wholesome foods. Engage in fun physical activities with them such as biking, swimming, playing ball, or walking at the zoo. Instead of using food as a reward substitute special outings, privileges, games or toys.

59. REALISTIC THOUGHTS

Our thoughts can get us into trouble when dieting. Be careful of all or nothing thinking in which you abstain completely from "bad" foods and eat only "good" foods. It is fine to eat all foods as long as you eat those with higher calories in limited amounts. The same applies to exercise. Plan for sensible exercise rather than extreme levels of exercise that you cannot sustain in the long run. That way you will not feel overwhelmed and give up. Be careful of "should" statements regarding food intake and exercise since these set you up for failure and a vicious cycle of bingeing, feeling bad about yourself, giving up, followed by even more unrealistic promises. If you aim for perfection you will set yourself up for failure. Aim for shades of gray in your thinking and you will keep moving forward with your plans.

60. BE OLD FASHIONED

Each generation is getting heavier than the previous one. Why is this happening? Food portions are considerably larger today than they were 20 years ago. The size of commonly eaten foods such as burgers, a portion of fries, or muffins has grown considerably. Beverage cups are also getting much larger. Additionally, we have more conveniences today designed to help us conserve energy. These include garage door openers, remote controls for television, numerous kitchen appliances, self-propelled vacuum cleaners, and dishwashers. If you want to lose weight switch to the smaller food portions you remember from your childhood. Get rid of the remote control for the TV and the garage door opener, wash dishes by hand instead of loading the dishwasher, do your own vacuuming, use an old-fashioned can opener, and mix your own batter instead of using a kitchen appliance for this. Every small lifestyle change helps.

61. BE PATIENT

It took you a long time to gain your weight, most likely years of eating more calories than you were burning. Recognize that it may now take some time to reverse this process and lose the weight that was accumulated over such a long period. Focus on the behavior changes you are making and on your weekly weight improvements. Before long you will be seeing noticeable differences when you look in a mirror. Remember, Rome was not built in a day. If you lose one to two pounds per week, that's a total of 52 to 104 pounds per year! Time will fly by if you stay on track and don't give up. Keep setting reachable, short-term goals to get you where you want to go. You could work on trying a new fruit, vegetable, or whole grain during the next week. Otherwise, you could sign up for an exercise class or try a new sport that you have always wanted to do. Show gratitude for all the small steps along the way.

62. WORK WITH YOUR GENES

Blaming your genes for your excess weight only keeps you a victim. Although genes determine your vulnerability to weight and body shape you are still the one making decisions regarding your lifestyle. If you change your eating and physical activity you will be able to break free from the family mold. You may have learned poor lifestyle habits from your family that support the notion that your weight problem is genetic. It's time to use your own personal power to take responsibility for your actions. You decide how much to eat and exercise, and you can carve out a completely different path for yourself. In the end, the effect of your environment is much greater than that of your genes in controlling your weight. You cannot do anything about your genes but you can do something about your environment. The best part is that you will be setting a great example for your kids and therefore ensuring a trimmer generation for the future.

63. FOCUS ON HEALTH

Lose weight for the sake of your health. That way, weight loss is something you're doing for your own benefit. You're taking care of yourself because you respect and care about your body. You want to make the right decisions in order to feel better and have more energy. By focusing on how great you feel when you're on track with your program you'll be less tempted to stray from your plan. You're not depriving yourself, you're looking after yourself. You're taking care of your heart and blood sugar levels, and reducing strain on your back and joints. You're also reducing your risk of developing cancer. You may sleep better at night and snore less. Weight loss may also improve your sex life. Imagine being able to run or climb stairs without getting out of breath. Imagine looking and feeling younger. It sure would be great to keep up with everyone else who's slim and trim. These healthy reasons make it all the more worthwhile to take care of your body. Remember, you're worth it.

64. SPEND TIME WITH HEALTHY PEOPLE

Have you ever noticed how easy it is to stay on track when you are with friends and family that have healthy lifestyles? They serve you wholesome food when you visit, make better food choices when eating out and suggest you go for a walk rather than watch TV. Since they rarely have a lot of junk food around, you are not constantly faced with temptation. Contrast this with how well you stay on track when spending time with people who have unhealthy lifestyles. You are continually bombarded with temptation as they snack on junk food and offer it to you. They cook unhealthy food and rarely engage in physical activity. If everyone around you is heavy it will seem more normal for you to also be heavy. One way to be successful is to surround yourself with successful people, and weight control is no exception. If you want an idea of how healthy you will be five years from now, look at the five people with whom you spend the most time today. Make a list of people who inspire you to be the best, healthiest person you can be and then spend more time with them.

65. REWARD JAR

We work much harder at something when we are rewarded for it, and weight loss is no exception. If you follow a behavior with a reward you increase the likelihood of doing that behavior again in the future. Therefore, you need to reward yourself for eating healthfully and exercising. Pick one goal for this project. For example, you may want to work on exercising more regularly. Get a jar and place it in a visible place in your home. Every time you exercise for at least 30 minutes, place a slip of paper in the jar. Write the date on the slip of paper and sign it. Before you start, determine a rate of exchange, for example, you pay yourself 50 cents for each slip of paper. The money can then be used to buy something that is very special and rewarding for you. If you like, you can get your significant other to chip in and help out, perhaps matching your reward dollar for dollar. You'll be surprised at how quickly you can accumulate slips of paper and get closer to your reward.

66. EAT REGULAR MEALS

Some people skip meals as a way to control weight. Often, they skip breakfast or eat very little for lunch. Their hunger usually builds up during the day, leaving them more likely to overeat later on. Unfortunately, the latter part of the day is not when you need to be consuming the majority of your calories. You are better off spreading out your calories during the entire day. Eat three healthy meals per day, plus a snack if you are hungry. The more you feel satisfied the less likely you are to give up on your plan and eat more than you need. If you are not a big breakfast eater try making a shake with low-fat milk, fresh fruit, and ice. It will kick-start your metabolism and leave you feeling more energized. Pack a healthy lunch for yourself, even fixing it the night before if necessary. That way you won't be tempted to miss out on it altogether. The trick is to provide your body with fuel throughout the day in order to keep your metabolism working full time.

67. YOU DON'T NEED MONEY TO LOSE WEIGHT

Weight loss does not have to be expensive. All you need is a comfortable pair of walking shoes and some healthy food. Unfortunately, a lot of diet, drug, and exercise companies would have you believe otherwise. They promote their own products, often accompanied by a weight loss guru who supposedly knows all the secrets to weight loss success. The secret is that there is no secret. All you need to do is eat fewer calories and move more. Therefore, you don't need to spend a lot of money to lose weight. You already have everything you need to get on track. In fact, falling prey to weight loss schemes may actually be more harmful to your health than simply being a few pounds overweight. The best proof of the fact that you don't need to spend money to lose weight is all the slim people in poor countries. Just remember that the next time you are being bombarded with an ad for yet another weight loss scheme.

68. WEIGHT CONTROL AS YOU GET OLDER

You often gain weight as you get older. This happens because you become less active and your metabolism slows down slightly. You also lose muscle mass, which originally helped you burn more calories. The best way to deal with these changes is to exercise and lift weights to burn calories and increase muscle mass. Anything you can do to remain active will help, even if exercising while seated. Swimming is a great sport for people of all ages. Although your appetite may not slow down, as you get older you need to make minor adjustments to your diet in order to consume fewer calories. Start gradually introducing healthier foods into your meals. Incorporating these changes into your lifestyle will actually benefit you twofold. In addition to keeping off excess weight, you will also be increasing your longevity. So, you get to be skinnier and live longer.

69. AVOID DIETS

Diets make you feel deprived. If you feel deprived you run the risk of eventually giving up and bingeing. Additionally, if you're on a diet sooner or later you will break it and resume your old eating habits. This applies especially to diets that make you give up an entire food group. You can do this for a short period but eventually will have to reintroduce this food back into your food plan. At that point you may regain all your weight. It is better to think about making reasonable lifestyle changes that are enduring. Think in terms of long-term commitments you can make rather than short-term gimmicks that will burn you out and give you yet another unsuccessful weight control experience. Stay focused on slow, steady means of getting your weight back on track. It's a better approach for both your physical and mental health.

70. EAT FROM A PLATE

Have you ever noticed that you eat more food if you eat it directly from a large container or serving plate? If the container is very large the food, in contrast, seems really small, leading us to eat more of it. Therefore, keep better track of what you are consuming by always eating from a plate on which you can see all the food. Additionally, if you get another serving of food keep your used plate on the table as a visual reminder of how much you have already eaten. If you keep removing plates from the table you'll have no idea how much food has already been consumed. This often happens at buffet restaurants or in all-you-can-eat situations. The same applies to free drink refills. After a while you have no idea how much of the drink you actually consumed. Avoid refills until you have finished your first glass of drink so you can keep track of your consumption. The more you know the better you can control your weight.

71. RECLAIM YOUR SALAD

We often view a salad as a healthy food item and a good choice when eating out. However, the healthy ingredients are often drowned with ingredients that can make your salad end up having more calories than expected. Most salads come covered with grated or cubed cheese, ham or bacon, adding both calories and fat. Tuna or egg "salads" contain a lot of mayonnaise. Fried croutons or noodles and some nuts or sunflower seeds add even more calories. Avocados, although good for you, add a lot of calories. Top the salad off with a thick dressing such as Ranch or blue cheese and your calorie count for your salad may well exceed that for a hamburger. To reclaim the nutritional benefits of your salad, use only fresh vegetables. Top off with a small serving of grilled chicken or salmon, if desired. Use a dressing of lemon juice or vinegar, herbs, and a small amount of olive oil. If you must use bottled dressing, use low-calorie dressing and dilute with water.

72. SPIRITUALITY MAY HELP

Many people have had success incorporating spirituality into their weight loss efforts. If you believe your body is a gift from a higher power you will want to treasure and respect it. You will also honor your body's built-in programming that tells you when you are hungry and full. The more you believe in your body's perfection the more you will focus inward and trust these signals. This new awareness will help you determine when and how much to eat. Some people have found prayer to be very helpful in staying on track. Believing that you are getting help from a higher source will keep you wanting to look after yourself. Asking for help and expressing gratitude for how far you have come can go a long way toward keeping you on track. Even more good news is that people who pray and meditate have lower blood pressure and a lower level of stress hormones, further adding to your health.

73. READ FOOD LABELS

Get in the habit of reading food labels in order to educate yourself about the nutritional values of different foods. For example, read labels from three or four different breakfast cereals at the same time. Determine which one is lowest in calories, total fat, saturated fat, trans fats, cholesterol and sodium. This would be your healthiest choice. Try to select items that also have a higher percent daily value of dietary fiber, vitamins and minerals. Food labels also tell you the proper serving size for each food item. Keep in mind that the serving sizes and percent daily values are based on consuming a 2,000-calorie per day diet. However, women and young children may need less calories and therefore smaller servings than this amount. People wishing to lose weight may also need less than this amount. Adolescents who are not trying to lose weight may actually need more than this amount.

74. RAISING NORMAL WEIGHT CHILDREN

It is best not to use food as a reward or punishment with children. Use non-food rewards such as special outings or privileges, time spent with favorite friends or family members, or small toys. Serve moderate portions, and refrain from over restriction since this may backfire and lead to your child sneaking food. Serve treats in controlled portions so your child realizes it is possible to eat fun foods as long as the quantities are reasonable. Teach your child to stop eating when full instead of encouraging him or her to clean his or her plate. For quick snacks place normal servings of food in zip lock bags that are easy to grab. Encourage your child to try new vegetables and fruit. Don't be discouraged if they do not like these immediately. It usually takes trying a new food numerous times before you get used to it, so just keep trying to reintroduce these foods every so often. Make sure you limit your child's screen time, i.e., total time spent watching television, on the computer, tablet, smartphone, or playing video games.

75. THIS BOOK IS YOUR FRIEND

Refer to this book often. It contains everything you need to know to lose weight and keep it off. Go back and reread a few pages every so often to stay on track. Remember, no one cares as much about your body as you should. You live in your body so you want to take care of it for a very long time to come. If you ever feel yourself slipping back to your old ways, revisit some of the things that helped you to lose weight. Keep doing all the things you learned in this book and you will have a lifetime of health and happiness. Share your new knowledge with those around you. Be the inspiration they need to get on track to a healthier life. Talk the talk and walk the walk. Best of luck in being the absolute best, healthiest version of yourself.